MAGNIFICENT

Meals

2025 CALENDAR

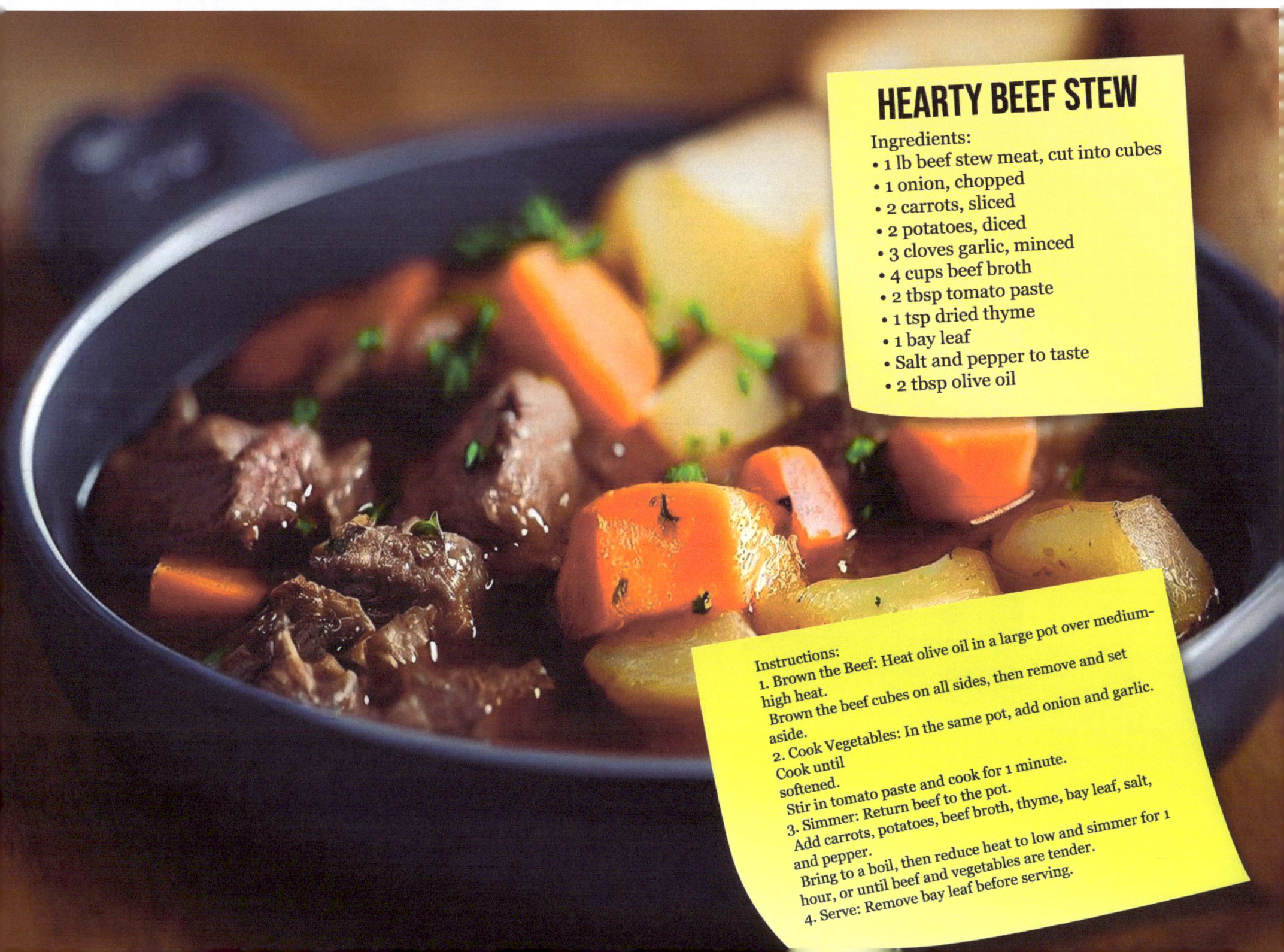

HEARTY BEEF STEW

Ingredients:
- 1 lb beef stew meat, cut into cubes
- 1 onion, chopped
- 2 carrots, sliced
- 2 potatoes, diced
- 3 cloves garlic, minced
- 4 cups beef broth
- 2 tbsp tomato paste
- 1 tsp dried thyme
- 1 bay leaf
- Salt and pepper to taste
- 2 tbsp olive oil

Instructions:
1. Brown the Beef: Heat olive oil in a large pot over medium-high heat.
Brown the beef cubes on all sides, then remove and set aside.
2. Cook Vegetables: In the same pot, add onion and garlic. Cook until softened.
Stir in tomato paste and cook for 1 minute.
3. Simmer: Return beef to the pot.
Add carrots, potatoes, beef broth, thyme, bay leaf, salt, and pepper.
Bring to a boil, then reduce heat to low and simmer for 1 hour, or until beef and vegetables are tender.
4. Serve: Remove bay leaf before serving.

JANUARY 2025

SUNDAY	MONDAY	TUESDAY	WEDNESDAY	THURSDAY	FRIDAY	SATURDAY
29	30	31	1	2	3	4
5	6	7	8	9	10	11
12	13	14	15	16	17	18
19	20	21	22	23	24	25
26	27	28	29	30	31	1

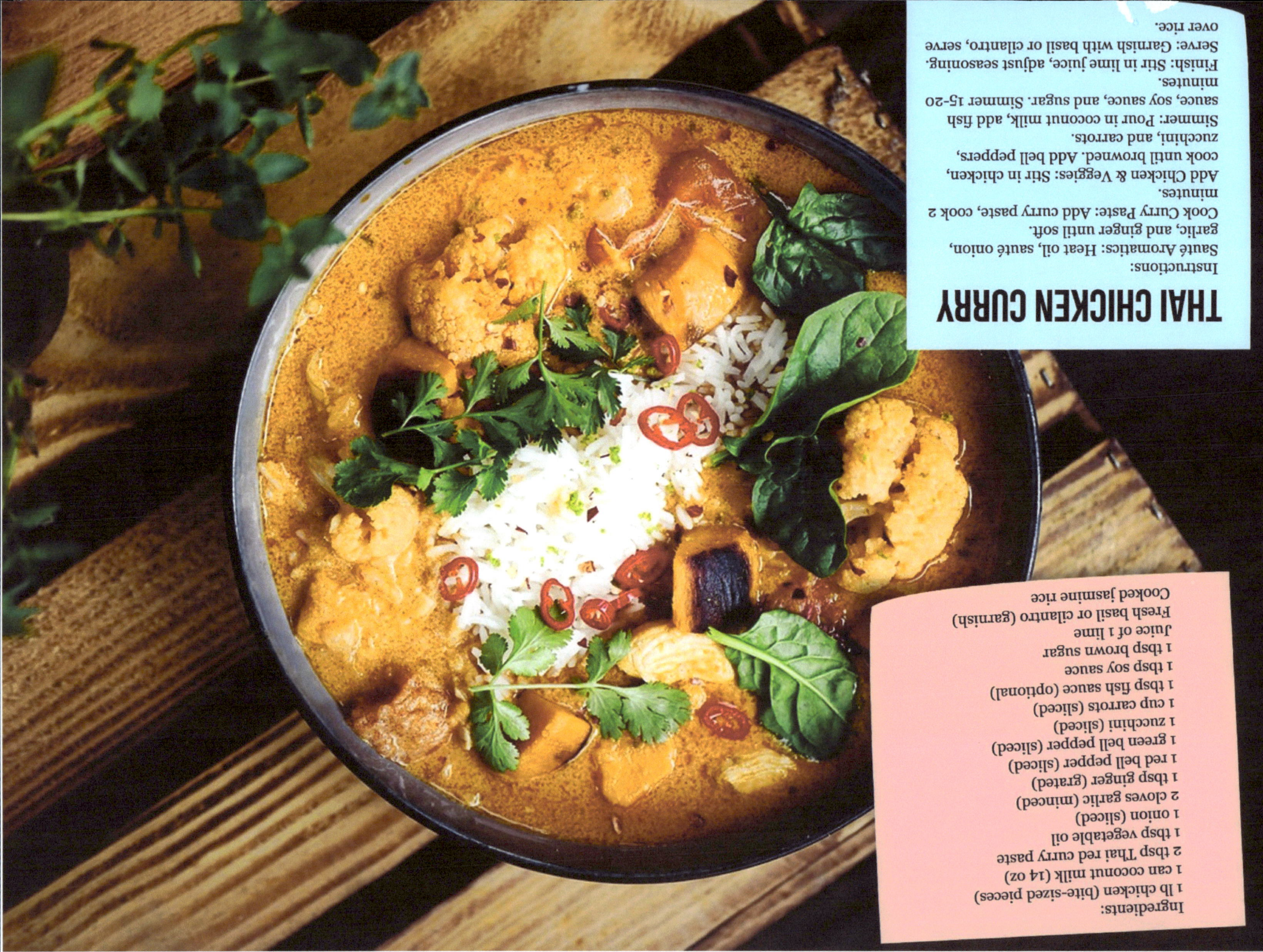

THAI CHICKEN CURRY

Instructions:

Sauté Aromatics: Heat oil, sauté onion, garlic, and ginger until soft.

Cook Curry Paste: Add curry paste, cook 2 minutes.

Add Chicken & Veggies: Stir in chicken, cook until browned. Add bell peppers, zucchini, and carrots.

Simmer: Pour in coconut milk, add fish sauce, soy sauce, and sugar. Simmer 15-20 minutes.

Finish: Stir in lime juice, adjust seasoning.

Serve: Garnish with basil or cilantro, serve over rice.

Ingredients:

1 lb chicken (bite-sized pieces)
1 can coconut milk (14 oz)
2 tbsp Thai red curry paste
1 tbsp vegetable oil
1 onion (sliced)
2 cloves garlic (minced)
1 tbsp ginger (grated)
1 red bell pepper (sliced)
1 green bell pepper (sliced)
1 zucchini (sliced)
1 cup carrots (sliced)
1 tbsp fish sauce (optional)
1 tbsp soy sauce
1 tbsp brown sugar
Juice of 1 lime
Fresh basil or cilantro (garnish)
Cooked jasmine rice

FEBRUARY 2025

SUNDAY	MONDAY	TUESDAY	WEDNESDAY	THURSDAY	FRIDAY	SATURDAY
26	27	28	29	30	31	1
2	3	4	5	6	7	8
9	10	11	12	13	14	15
16	17	18	19	20	21	22
23	24	25	26	27	28	1

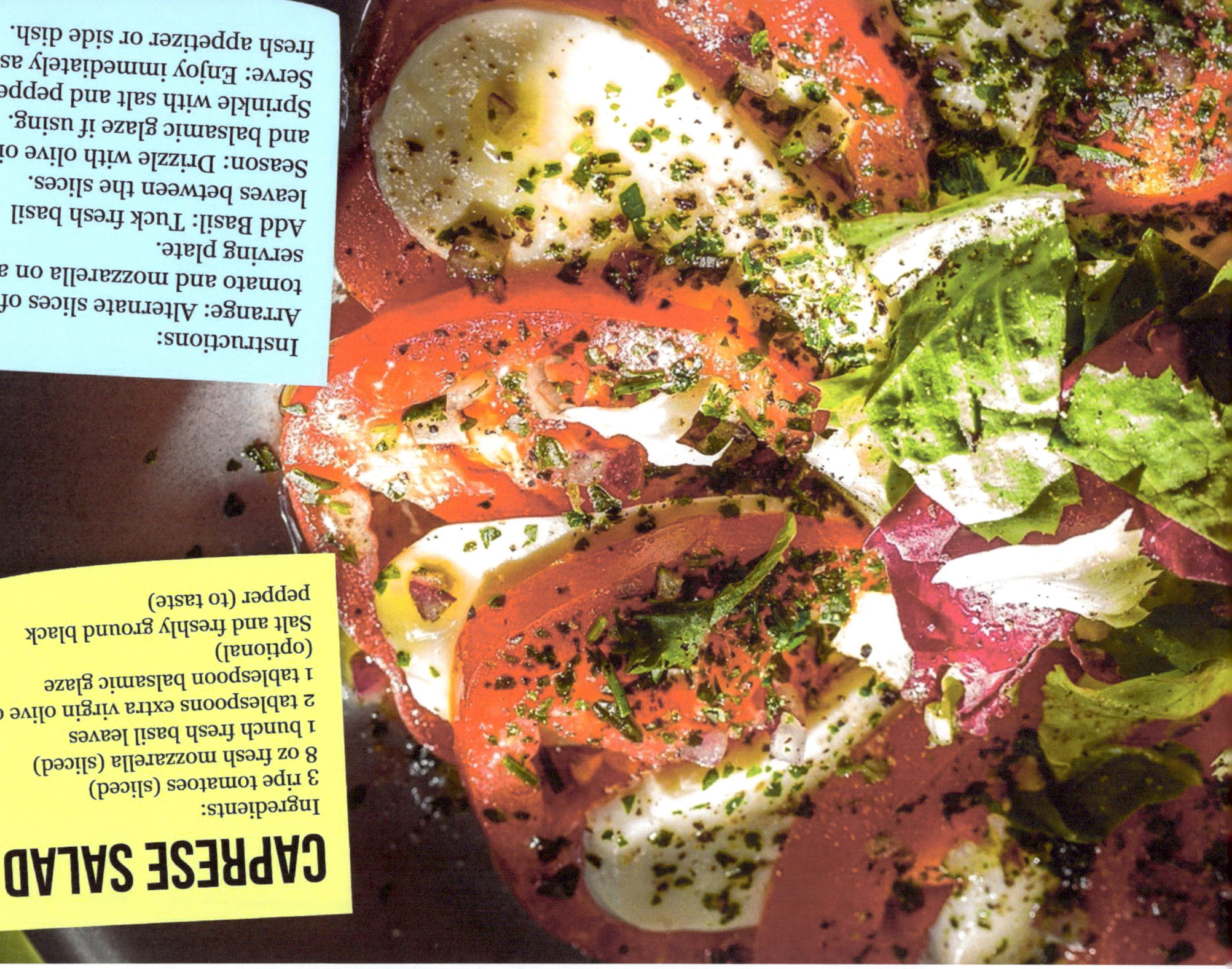

CAPRESE SALAD

Ingredients:
3 ripe tomatoes (sliced)
8 oz fresh mozzarella (sliced)
1 bunch fresh basil leaves
2 tablespoons extra virgin olive oil
1 tablespoon balsamic glaze (optional)
Salt and freshly ground black pepper (to taste)

Instructions:
Arrange: Alternate slices of tomato and mozzarella on a serving plate.
Add Basil: Tuck fresh basil leaves between the slices.
Season: Drizzle with olive oil and balsamic glaze if using. Sprinkle with salt and pepper.
Serve: Enjoy immediately as a fresh appetizer or side dish.

MARCH 2025

SUNDAY	MONDAY	TUESDAY	WEDNESDAY	THURSDAY	FRIDAY	SATURDAY
23	24	25	26	27	28	1
2	3	4	5	6	7	8
9	10	11	12	13	14	15
16	17	18	19	20	21	22
23 / 30	24 / 31	25	26	27	28	29

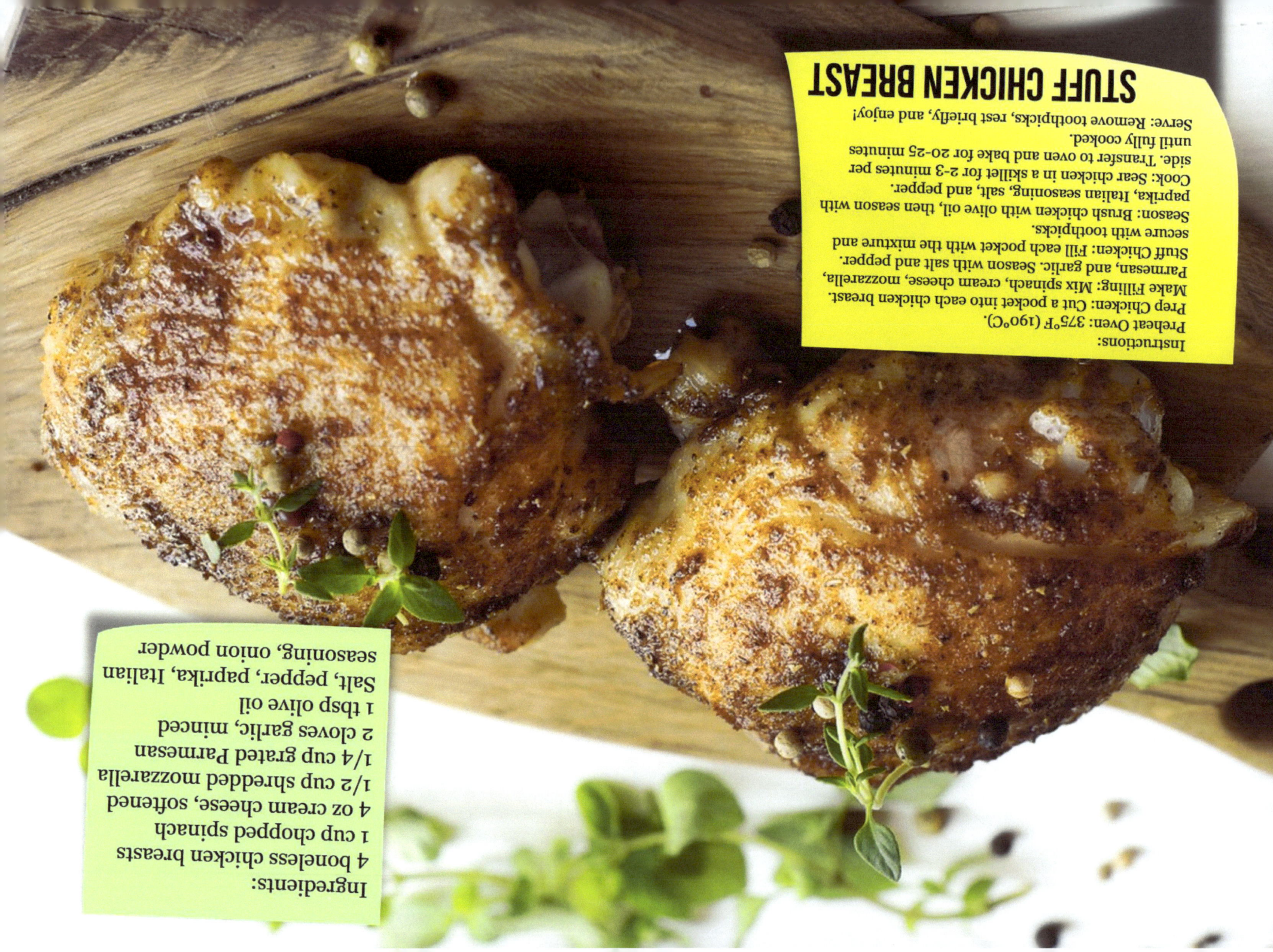

STUFF CHICKEN BREAST

Instructions:
Preheat Oven: 375°F (190°C).
Prep Chicken: Cut a pocket into each chicken breast.
Make Filling: Mix spinach, cream cheese, mozzarella, Parmesan, and garlic. Season with salt and pepper.
Stuff Chicken: Fill each pocket with the mixture and secure with toothpicks.
Season: Brush chicken with olive oil, then season with paprika, Italian seasoning, salt, and pepper.
Cook: Sear chicken in a skillet for 2-3 minutes per side. Transfer to oven and bake for 20-25 minutes until fully cooked.
Serve: Remove toothpicks, rest briefly, and enjoy!

Ingredients:
4 boneless chicken breasts
1 cup chopped spinach
4 oz cream cheese, softened
1/2 cup shredded mozzarella
1/4 cup grated Parmesan
2 cloves garlic, minced
1 tbsp olive oil
Salt, pepper, paprika, Italian seasoning, onion powder

APRIL 2025

SUNDAY	MONDAY	TUESDAY	WEDNESDAY	THURSDAY	FRIDAY	SATURDAY
30	31	1	2	3	4	5
6	7	8	9	10	11	12
13	14	15	16	17	18	19
20	21	22	23	24	25	26
27	28	29	30	1	2	3

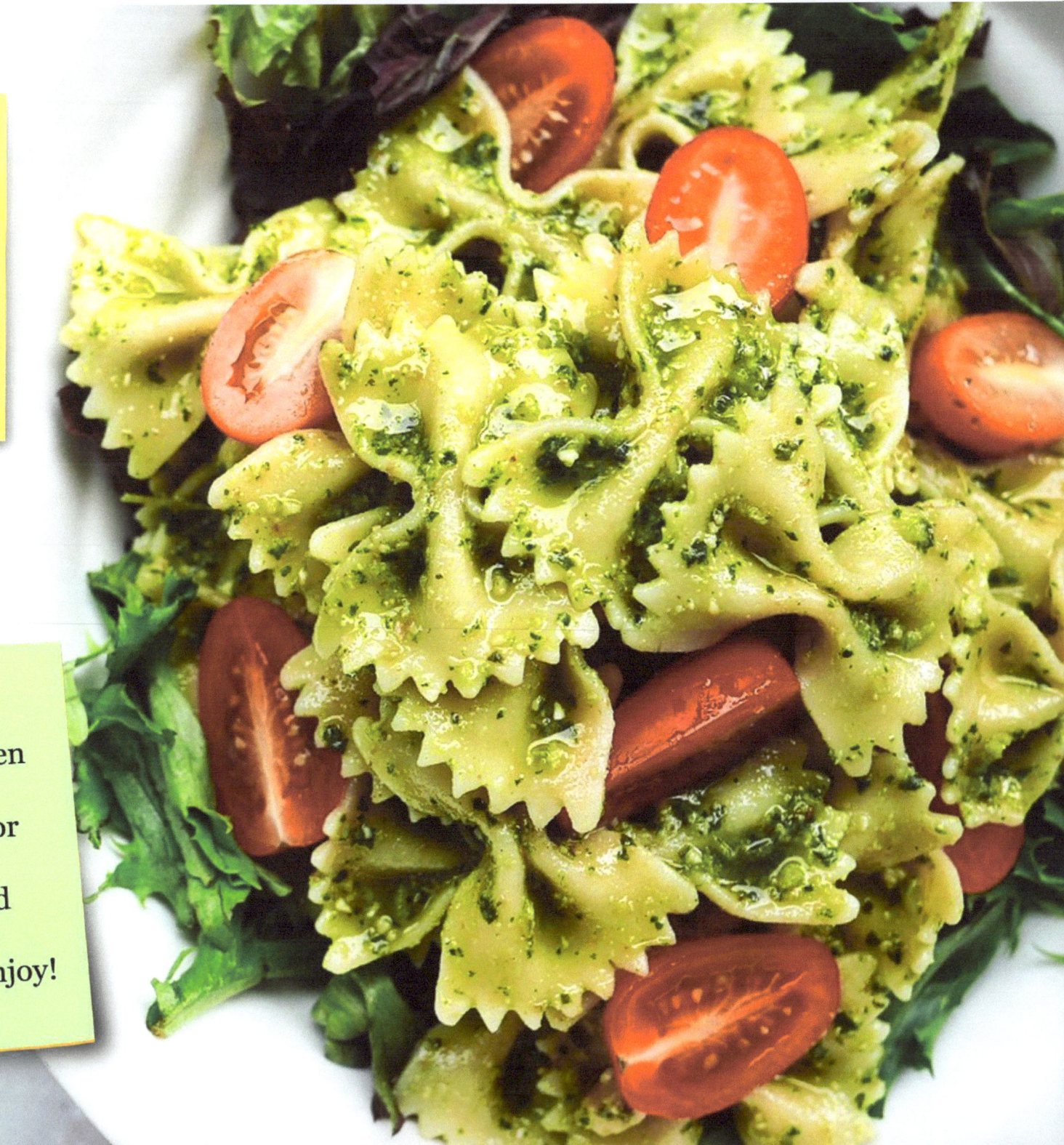

BOW TIE PESTO PASTA

Ingredients:
12 oz bow tie pasta
1 cup cherry tomatoes, halved
1/2 cup pesto sauce
1/4 cup grated Parmesan
2 tbsp olive oil
Salt and pepper

Instructions:
Cook pasta until al dente, then drain.
Sauté tomatoes in olive oil for 2-3 minutes.
Mix pasta with tomatoes and pesto in the skillet. Season.
Serve with Parmesan and enjoy!

MAY 2025

SUNDAY	MONDAY	TUESDAY	WEDNESDAY	THURSDAY	FRIDAY	SATURDAY
27	28	29	30	1	2	3
4	5	6	7	8	9	10
11	12	13	14	15	16	17
18	19	20	21	22	23	24
25	26	27	28	29	30	31

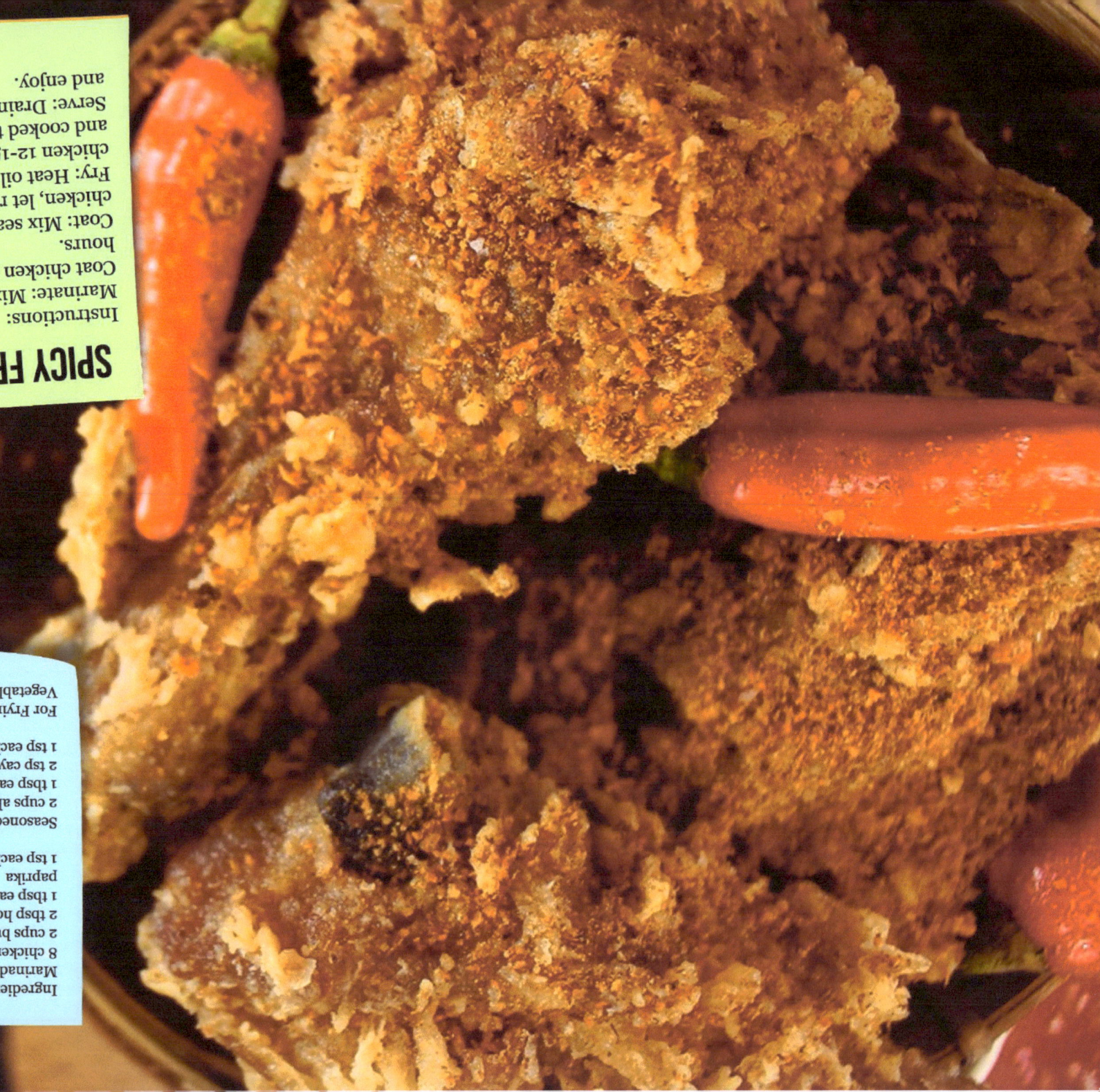

SPICY FRIED CHICKEN

Instructions:
Marinate: Mix marinade ingredients. Coat chicken and refrigerate 4+ hours.
Coat: Mix seasoned flour. Dredge chicken, let rest 15 minutes.
Fry: Heat oil to 350°F (175°C). Fry chicken 12-15 minutes until golden and cooked through.
Serve: Drain on paper towels, let rest, and enjoy.

Ingredients:
Marinade:
8 chicken pieces (thighs and drumsticks)
2 cups buttermilk
2 tbsp hot sauce
1 tbsp each: garlic powder, onion powder, paprika
1 tsp each: cayenne pepper, salt, black pepper

Seasoned Flour:
2 cups all-purpose flour
1 tbsp each: paprika, garlic powder, onion powder
2 tsp cayenne pepper
1 tsp each: salt, black pepper, oregano, thyme

For Frying:
Vegetable or peanut oil

JUNE 2025

SUNDAY	MONDAY	TUESDAY	WEDNESDAY	THURSDAY	FRIDAY	SATURDAY
1	2	3	4	5	6	7
8	9	10	11	12	13	14
15	16	17	18	19	20	21
22	23	24	25	26	27	28
29	30	1	2	3	4	5

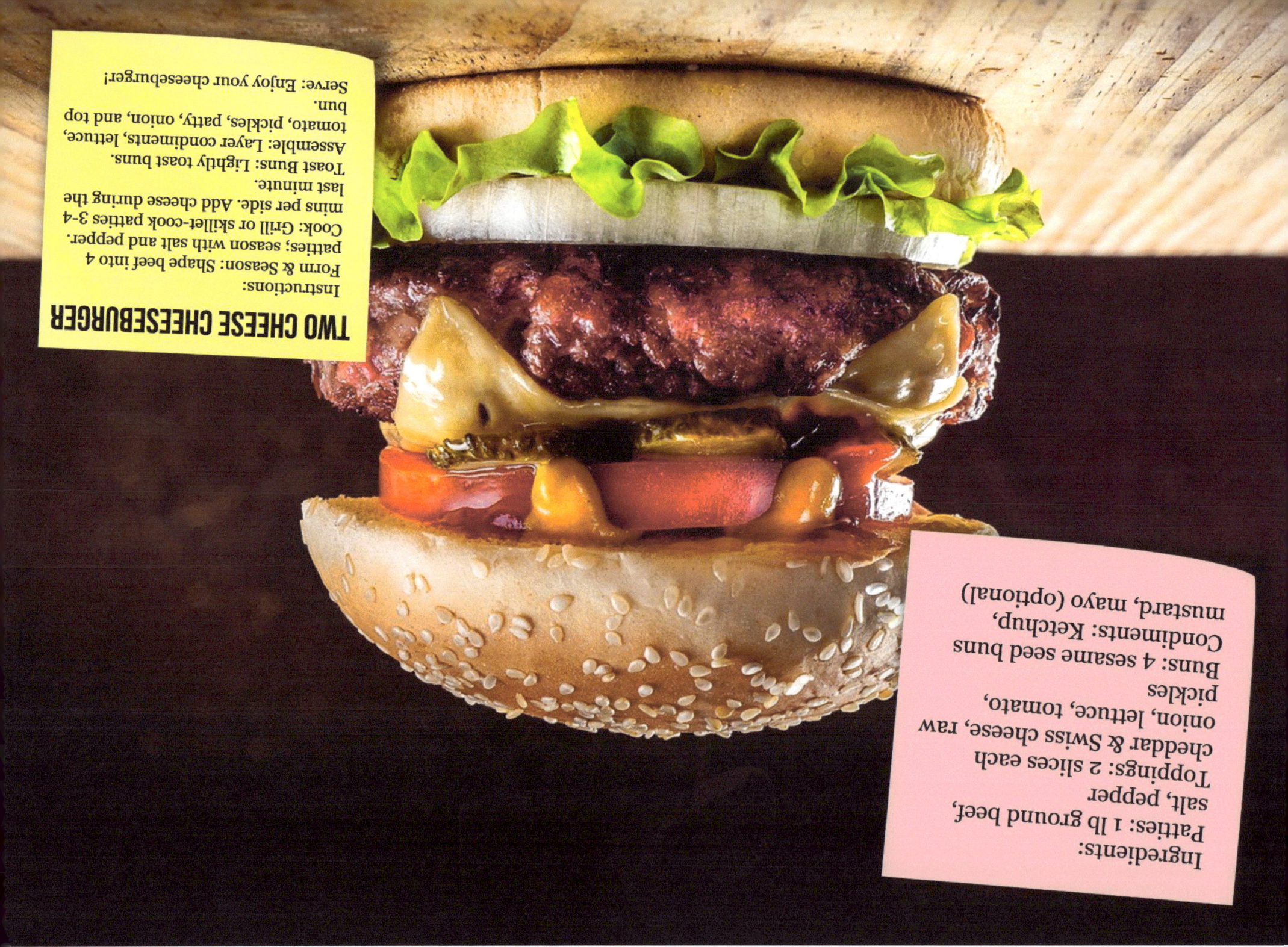

TWO CHEESEBURGER

Instructions:
Form & Season: Shape beef into 4 patties; season with salt and pepper.
Cook: Grill or skillet-cook patties 3-4 mins per side. Add cheese during the last minute.
Toast Buns: Lightly toast buns.
Assemble: Layer condiments, lettuce, tomato, pickles, patty, onion, and top bun.
Serve: Enjoy your cheeseburger!

Ingredients:
Patties: 1 lb ground beef, salt, pepper
Toppings: 2 slices each cheddar & Swiss cheese, raw onion, lettuce, tomato, pickles
Buns: 4 sesame seed buns
Condiments: Ketchup, mustard, mayo (optional)

JULY 2025

SUNDAY	MONDAY	TUESDAY	WEDNESDAY	THURSDAY	FRIDAY	SATURDAY
29	30	1	2	3	4	5
6	7	8	9	10	11	12
13	14	15	16	17	18	19
20	21	22	23	24	25	26
27	28	29	30	31	1	2

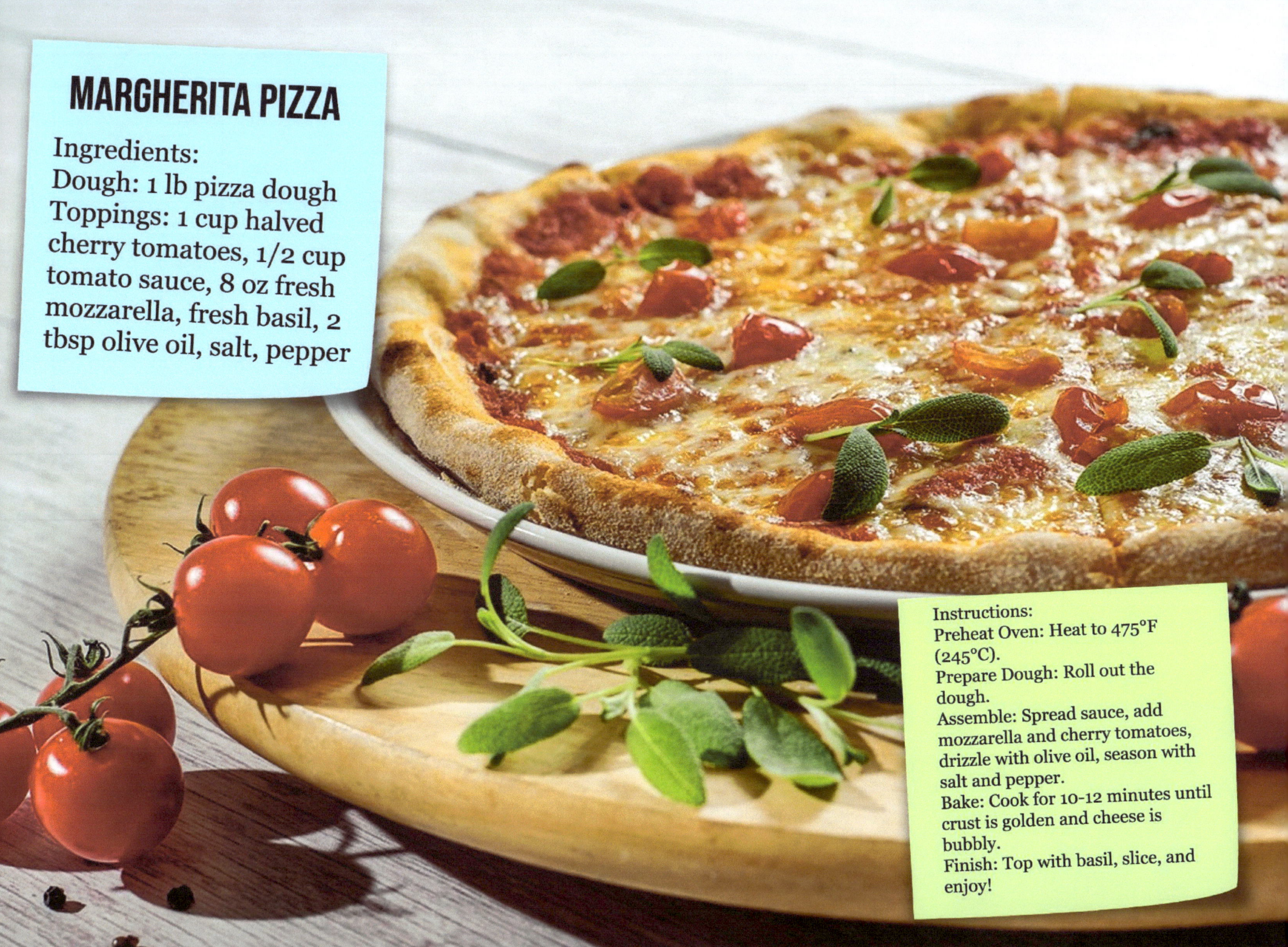

MARGHERITA PIZZA

Ingredients:
Dough: 1 lb pizza dough
Toppings: 1 cup halved cherry tomatoes, 1/2 cup tomato sauce, 8 oz fresh mozzarella, fresh basil, 2 tbsp olive oil, salt, pepper

Instructions:
Preheat Oven: Heat to 475°F (245°C).
Prepare Dough: Roll out the dough.
Assemble: Spread sauce, add mozzarella and cherry tomatoes, drizzle with olive oil, season with salt and pepper.
Bake: Cook for 10-12 minutes until crust is golden and cheese is bubbly.
Finish: Top with basil, slice, and enjoy!

AUGUST 2025

SUNDAY	MONDAY	TUESDAY	WEDNESDAY	THURSDAY	FRIDAY	SATURDAY
27	28	29	30	31	1	2
3	4	5	6	7	8	9
10	11	12	13	14	15	16
17	18	19	20	21	22	23
24 / 31	25	26	27	28	29	30

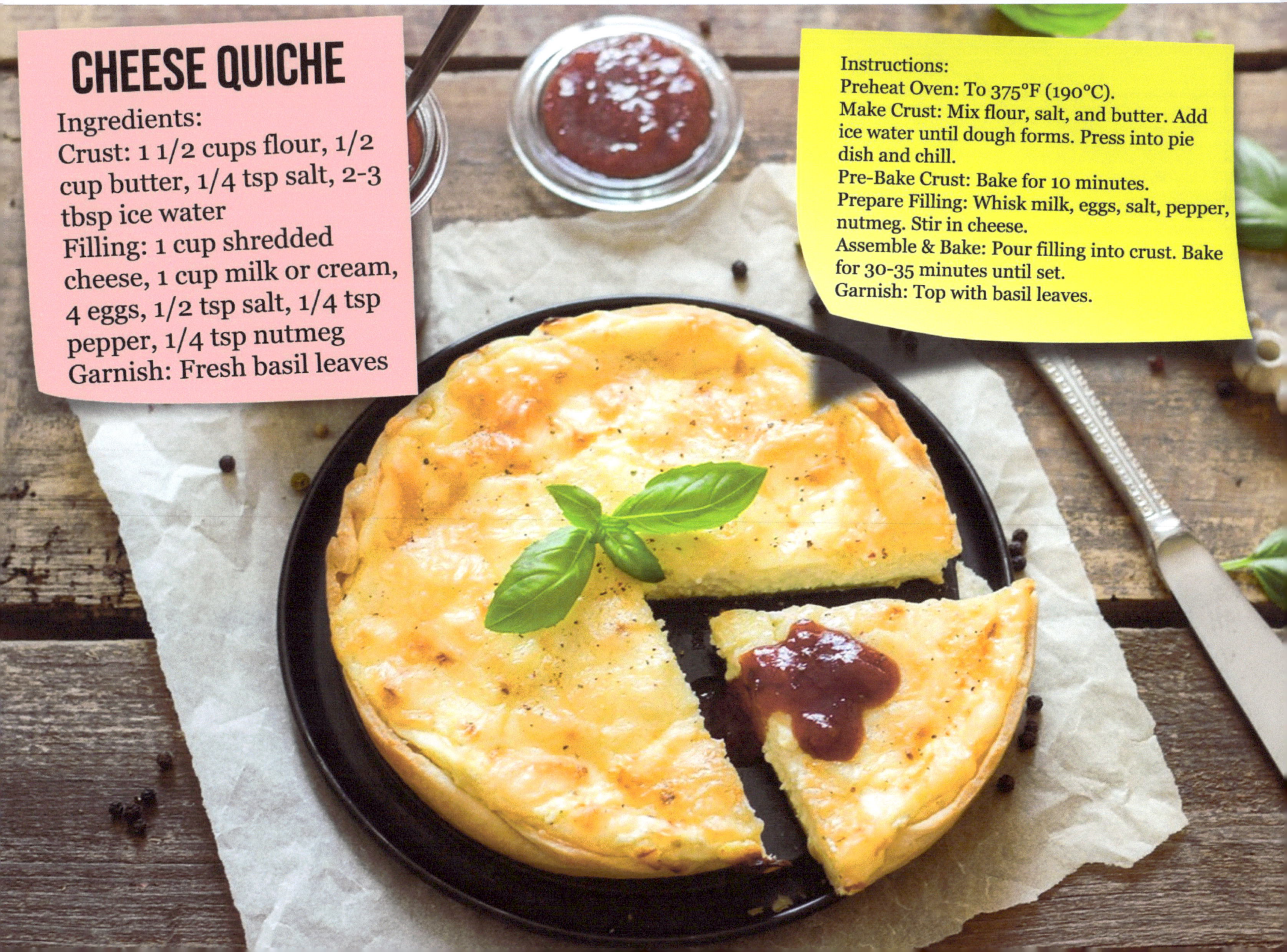

CHEESE QUICHE

Ingredients:
Crust: 1 1/2 cups flour, 1/2 cup butter, 1/4 tsp salt, 2-3 tbsp ice water
Filling: 1 cup shredded cheese, 1 cup milk or cream, 4 eggs, 1/2 tsp salt, 1/4 tsp pepper, 1/4 tsp nutmeg
Garnish: Fresh basil leaves

Instructions:
Preheat Oven: To 375°F (190°C).
Make Crust: Mix flour, salt, and butter. Add ice water until dough forms. Press into pie dish and chill.
Pre-Bake Crust: Bake for 10 minutes.
Prepare Filling: Whisk milk, eggs, salt, pepper, nutmeg. Stir in cheese.
Assemble & Bake: Pour filling into crust. Bake for 30-35 minutes until set.
Garnish: Top with basil leaves.

SEPTEMBER 2025

SUNDAY	MONDAY	TUESDAY	WEDNESDAY	THURSDAY	FRIDAY	SATURDAY
31	1	2	3	4	5	6
7	8	9	10	11	12	13
14	15	16	17	18	19	20
21	22	23	24	25	26	27
28	29	30	1	2	3	4

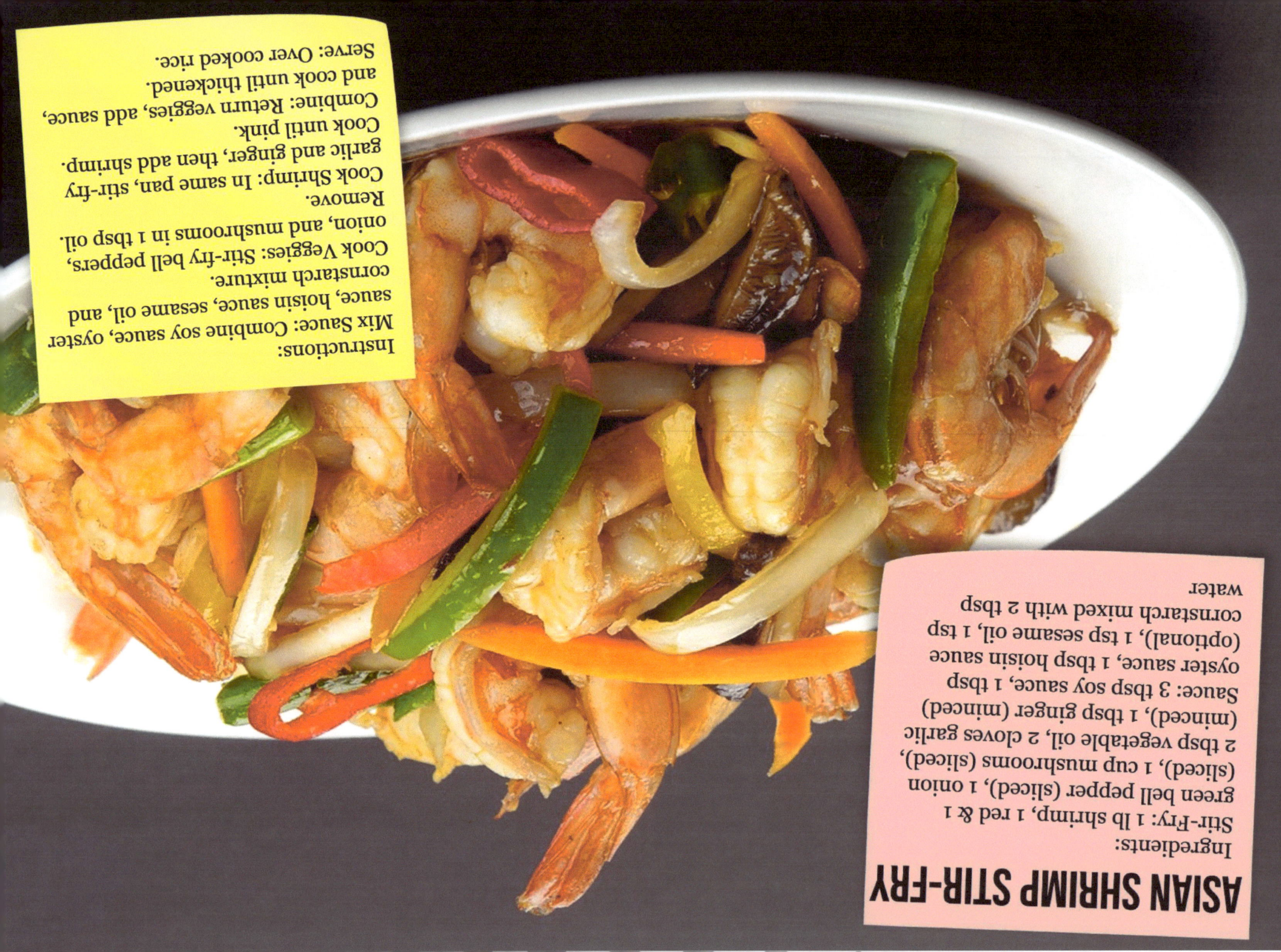

ASIAN SHRIMP STIR-FRY

Ingredients:

Stir-Fry: 1 lb shrimp, 1 red & 1 green bell pepper (sliced), 1 onion (sliced), 1 cup mushrooms (sliced), 2 tbsp vegetable oil, 2 cloves garlic (minced), 1 tbsp ginger (minced)

Sauce: 3 tbsp soy sauce, 1 tbsp oyster sauce, 1 tbsp hoisin sauce (optional), 1 tsp sesame oil, 1 tsp cornstarch mixed with 2 tbsp water

Instructions:

Mix Sauce: Combine soy sauce, oyster sauce, hoisin sauce, sesame oil, and cornstarch mixture.

Cook Veggies: Stir-fry bell peppers, onion, and mushrooms in 1 tbsp oil. Remove.

Cook Shrimp: In same pan, stir-fry garlic and ginger, then add shrimp. Cook until pink.

Combine: Return veggies, add sauce, and cook until thickened.

Serve: Over cooked rice.

OCTOBER 2025

SUNDAY	MONDAY	TUESDAY	WEDNESDAY	THURSDAY	FRIDAY	SATURDAY
28	29	30	1	2	3	4
5	6	7	8	9	10	11
12	13	14	15	16	17	18
19	20	21	22	23	24	25
26	27	28	29	30	31	1

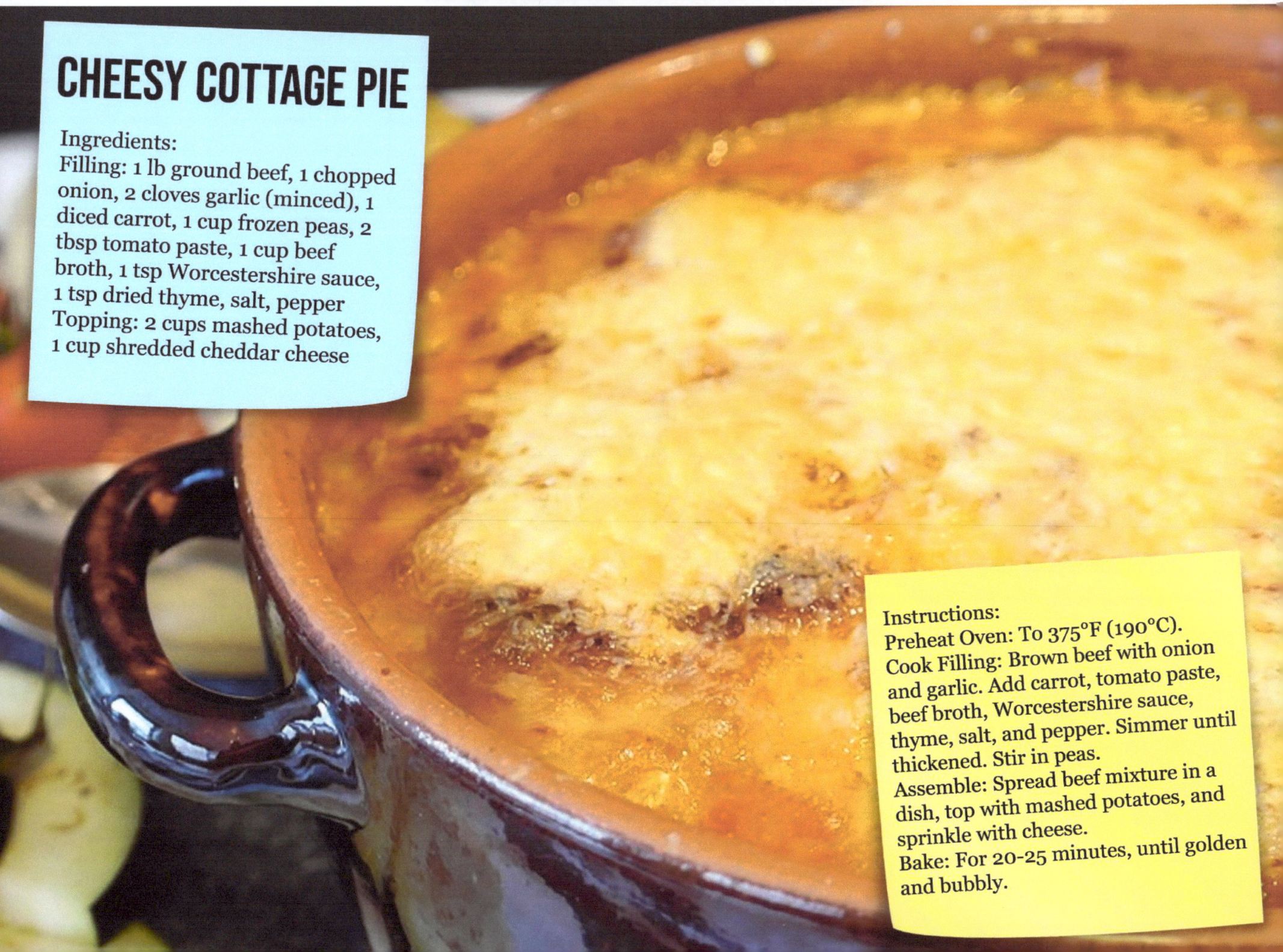

CHEESY COTTAGE PIE

Ingredients:
Filling: 1 lb ground beef, 1 chopped onion, 2 cloves garlic (minced), 1 diced carrot, 1 cup frozen peas, 2 tbsp tomato paste, 1 cup beef broth, 1 tsp Worcestershire sauce, 1 tsp dried thyme, salt, pepper
Topping: 2 cups mashed potatoes, 1 cup shredded cheddar cheese

Instructions:
Preheat Oven: To 375°F (190°C).
Cook Filling: Brown beef with onion and garlic. Add carrot, tomato paste, beef broth, Worcestershire sauce, thyme, salt, and pepper. Simmer until thickened. Stir in peas.
Assemble: Spread beef mixture in a dish, top with mashed potatoes, and sprinkle with cheese.
Bake: For 20-25 minutes, until golden and bubbly.

NOVEMBER 2025

SUNDAY	MONDAY	TUESDAY	WEDNESDAY	THURSDAY	FRIDAY	SATURDAY
26	27	28	29	30	31	1
2	3	4	5	6	7	8
9	10	11	12	13	14	15
16	17	18	19	20	21	22
23 / 30	24	25	26	27	28	29

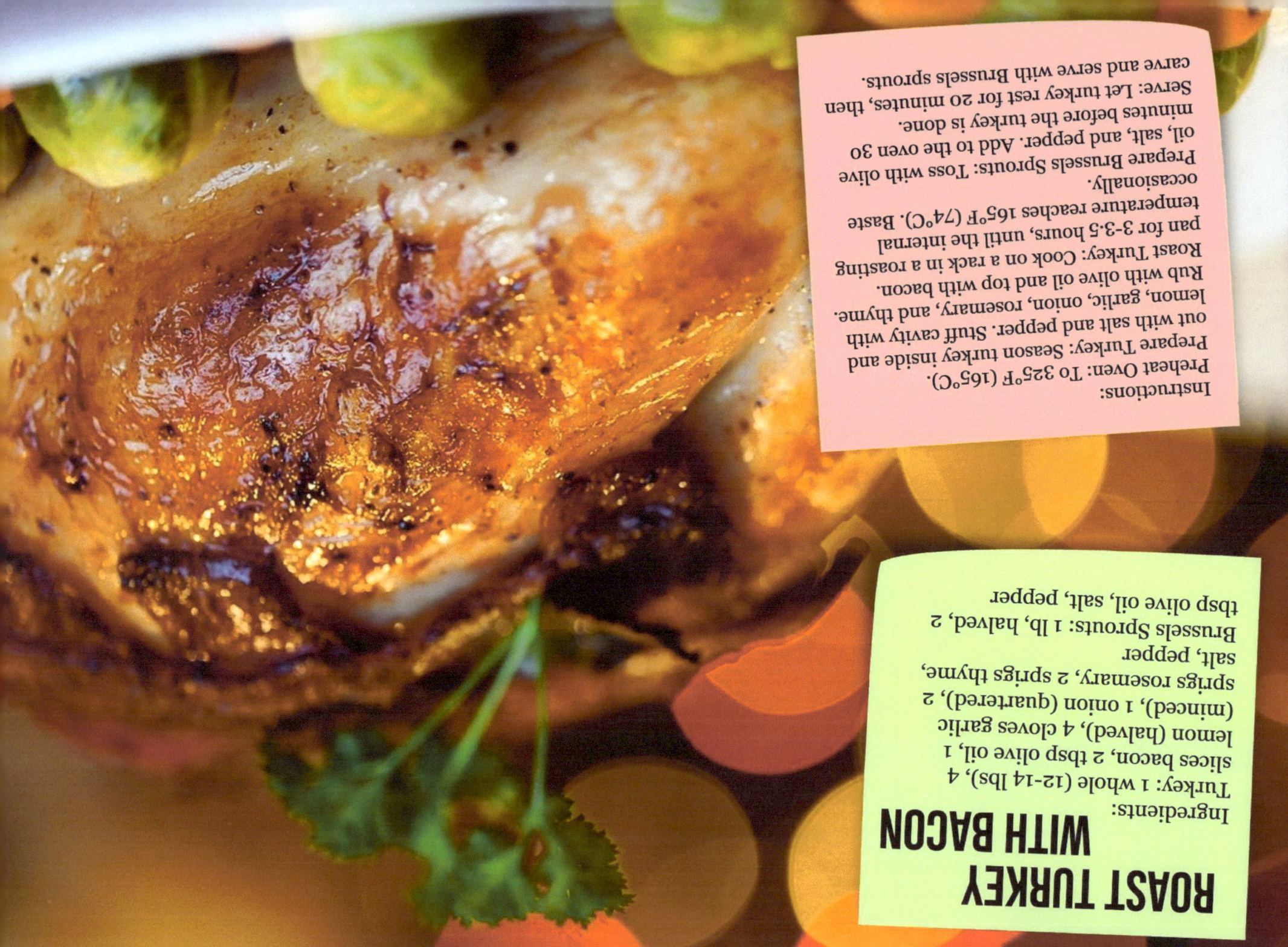

ROAST TURKEY WITH BACON

Ingredients:
Turkey: 1 whole (12-14 lbs), 4 slices bacon, 2 tbsp olive oil, 1 lemon (halved), 4 cloves garlic (minced), 1 onion (quartered), 2 sprigs rosemary, 2 sprigs thyme, salt, pepper
Brussels Sprouts: 1 lb, halved, 2 tbsp olive oil, salt, pepper

Instructions:
Preheat Oven: To 325°F (165°C).
Prepare Turkey: Season turkey inside and out with salt and pepper. Stuff cavity with lemon, garlic, onion, rosemary, and thyme. Rub with olive oil and top with bacon.
Roast Turkey: Cook on a rack in a roasting pan for 3-3.5 hours, until the internal temperature reaches 165°F (74°C). Baste occasionally.
Prepare Brussels Sprouts: Toss with olive oil, salt, and pepper. Add to the oven 30 minutes before the turkey is done.
Serve: Let turkey rest for 20 minutes, then carve and serve with Brussels sprouts.

DECEMBER 2025

SUNDAY	MONDAY	TUESDAY	WEDNESDAY	THURSDAY	FRIDAY	SATURDAY
30	1	2	3	4	5	6
7	8	9	10	11	12	13
14	15	16	17	18	19	20
21	22	23	24	25	26	27
28	29	30	31	1	2	3

DESSERTS

January: Warm Apple Crisp
Description: Cozy and comforting, apple crisp is perfect for chilly winter days. Baked apples topped with a crunchy oat and cinnamon crumble.
Ingredients: Apples, oats, flour, butter, brown sugar, cinnamon.
Instructions: Slice apples, mix with cinnamon and sugar. Top with oat mixture and bake until golden.

February: Chocolate Lava Cake
Description: Rich, gooey chocolate cake with a molten center, ideal for Valentine's Day indulgence.
Ingredients: Dark chocolate, butter, eggs, sugar, flour.
Instructions: Melt chocolate and butter, mix with other ingredients, bake until the edges are set and the center is molten.

March: Lemon Bars
Description: Tangy and sweet, lemon bars are a bright way to welcome spring. A buttery shortbread crust topped with a zesty lemon filling.
Ingredients: Lemons, sugar, eggs, flour, butter.
Instructions: Bake shortbread crust, pour lemon mixture over, bake again until set.

April: Carrot Cake
Description: Moist and spiced, carrot cake with cream cheese frosting is perfect for springtime celebrations.
Ingredients: Carrots, flour, sugar, eggs, cinnamon, cream cheese.
Instructions: Mix grated carrots with other ingredients, bake, and top with cream cheese frosting.

May: Strawberry Shortcake
Description: Fresh strawberries layered with sweet biscuits and whipped cream, capturing the essence of spring.
Ingredients: Strawberries, sugar, flour, butter, cream.
Instructions: Bake biscuits, slice strawberries, and layer with whipped cream.

June: Key Lime Pie
Description: Tart and creamy, key lime pie is a refreshing dessert for early summer.
Ingredients: Key lime juice, sweetened condensed milk, graham cracker crust, eggs.
Instructions: Mix key lime juice with condensed milk and eggs, pour into crust, and bake.

July: Mixed Berry Pavlova
Description: Light and airy meringue topped with whipped cream and a mix of summer berries.
Ingredients: Egg whites, sugar, cream, assorted berries.
Instructions: Bake meringue until crisp, top with whipped cream and fresh berries.

August: Peach Cobbler
Description: Juicy peaches baked with a fluffy biscuit topping, perfect for late summer.
Ingredients: Peaches, sugar, flour, butter, baking powder.
Instructions: Toss peaches with sugar, top with biscuit dough, and bake until golden.

September: Fig and Almond Tart
Description: A delicate tart with sweet figs and almond cream, celebrating the flavors of early fall.
Ingredients: Fresh figs, almonds, butter, sugar, flour.
Instructions: Make almond cream, fill tart shell, top with figs, and bake.

October: Pumpkin Pie
Description: Classic pumpkin pie with warm spices, a must-have for autumn gatherings.
Ingredients: Pumpkin puree, eggs, sugar, cinnamon, nutmeg, pie crust.
Instructions: Mix pumpkin with spices and eggs, pour into crust, and bake until set.

November: Pecan Pie
Description: Rich and nutty, pecan pie is a staple for Thanksgiving celebrations.
Ingredients: Pecans, corn syrup, sugar, eggs, butter, pie crust.
Instructions: Mix pecans with filling, pour into crust, and bake until set.

December: Gingerbread Cookies
Description: Spiced gingerbread cookies, perfect for holiday decorating and sharing.
Ingredients: Ginger, cinnamon, flour, sugar, butter, molasses.
Instructions: Mix dough, chill, roll out, cut shapes, and bake. Decorate with icing.